The
Healing Power
of
God

Prophetess Carolyn Jones Powe

ISBN:
978-0-578-79389-4

DEDICATION

To my loving husband, Apostle Lesley Powe, who serves as a light to help lead me in the path, destiny, and purpose that God has preordained for my life. To my daughter, LaKeshia Sherell Powe, whose moral strength and tenacity enables her to resist opposition and remain persistent in reaching set goals.

CONTENT

ACKNOWLEDGMENTS

First, I would like to Thank God for giving me divine insight on His Word concerning His limitless healing power and His guidance in writing this book. I wish to acknowledge the many people whom I have met throughout the years that have served as an inspiration to me. Also, I wish to acknowledge Gloria McGrew Everett for helping me complete this project. As I stayed in the presence of God, I learned more and more about His healing power. At the time, I did not realize that God's Word carried the very power that I would need for my own healing deliverance. He sent His Word and healed me after the doctors had done everything medically possible for me. They gave up on me and gave me two weeks to live. That is when God sent His Word (Psalm 118:17) I shall not die, but live, and declare the works of the Lord.

INTRODUCTION

THE MIRACLE WORKING POWER OF GOD

This book on the healing power of God will serve as a resource of scriptural based information and personal healing testimonies as well. First and foremost, it is important that it be acknowledged that God's healing power is available to everyone who has faith and believes.

"In the book of Isaiah 55:11, it reads;

> *So is my word that goes out of my mouth: It will not return to me empty, but will accomplish what I desire and achieve The purpose for which I sent it."*

This book is written to enlighten people on the fact that God is the only source of hope for man, whether it be for healing, or deliverances of any nature. God is awesome in the way that He meticulously created and designed the human body. The word meticulous describes the way that God gave great attention to His creation of man. This word is very significant as used in this introduction. It means taking or showing extreme care about minute details. Because of God's

"Omnipotence", which means that God has unlimited authority and infinite power. He foresaw the health issues that man's body would encounter and made provision for it. God alone was the master architect in all of creation. There is a precious verse in Psalm 139:14 that says "I will praise Thee; for I am fearfully and wonderfully made; Marvelous are Thy works; and that my soul knoweth right well.

In the Old Testament God promised to take away sickness and disease as a result of man's continued obedience to His Word; (Exodus 15:26). The verse ended with, "For I am the Lord that healeth thee. In Deuteronomy 28; God healed everyone, so that there was not a sick person in all of the twelve tribes.

Also God made a special covenant with the children of Israel in Exodus 15:26 which says:

> *"And said, if thou wilt diligently hearken to the voice Of the Lord Thy God and will do that which is*
> *Right in His sight, and will give ear to His commandments*
> *And keep all of His statutes, I will put none of these diseases*
> *Upon thee, which I have brought upon the Egyptians: For I Am the Lord that healeth thee."*

Later in the New Testament. God sent His only Begotten Son to the children of this generation to confirm His word concerning The Healing Power of God. The power of God to heal is as effective today as it ever was. As one reads and studies the Word of God , your faith will begin to grow and become more active. In many instances Jesus told those that He healed that their faith had made them whole.

We are to glorify God in our body. 1 Corinthians 6:20 tells us plainly that "For ye are bought with a price; therefore glorify God in your body, and in your spirit which are God's."

CHAPTER 1

THE PHYSICAL MAKEUP OF THE HUMAN BODY

Chapter one deals with a brief description of the unique physical make-up of the human body.

"The human brain is the control center, which receives and sends signals to other organs throughout the nervous system. The brain is responsible for our thoughts, feelings, and memory storage as well as how many views and maintains life here on earth."

The human body has five vital organs that are essential for survival. They are as follows:

1. The Brain
2. The Heart
3. The Kidneys
4. The Liver
5. The Lungs

There are basic parts of the body which include:

1. The Head
2. The Neck
3. The Torso
4. The Arms

5.   The Legs

The body consists of a number of biological systems that carry out specific functions. These systems assist us in carrying out daily activities. The human body is uniquely ,created and designed. The body is not merely created to function in the natural, but also in the spiritual realm as well. In addition, the spirit is one of the sources of power and control for both your body and soul. According to 1 Corinthians 6:19 (KJV) it says, "What? Know ye not that your body is the temple of the Holy Ghost which is in you.

THE SPIRITUAL DESIGN OF THE HUMAN BODY

The Holy Spirit of God is the source of power and control for both, your body and soul: We are to glorify God in our body. 1st. Corinthians 6:20 describes plainly ; "For ye are bought with a price, therefore glorify God in your body and in your spirit, which are God's.
It is necessary that this writing deals with the spiritual design of the body as well as the physical design. The Lord originally designed man's body to be disease free by continuously living in divine health. He also made it possible for man's divine healing of any and all infirmities that attack the body by having faith in the healing power of God.
In the old testament , in the book of Exodus chapter 23 and verse 25, (KJV) And ye shall serve the Lord your God, and He shall bless thy bread and thy water; and I will take sickness away from the midst of thee."1st Peter 1:24 makes it quite clear that our

healing has already been completed or paid for by the stripes of Jesus Christ. The scripture says, "Who His own self bare our sins in His own body on the tree, that we, being dead to sins, should live unto righteousness, by whose stripes ye were healed. According to this verse, healing can be taken by faith in the word of God.

CHAPTER 2

THE BODY WAS DESIGNED TO HEAL ITSELF

Chapter two attempts to bring credence to the body's self-healing process.

There are many questions that concern people about the body's ability to heal itself. How do we tap into this process that allows the body to reap such an amazing benefit? The Lord was specific in the design of just how the body would function by the process of divine healing and divine health. But how do we walk in divine health? First of all, God in His infinite wisdom and creative power made the human body and placed within them the ability to heal themselves. For example, if you cut your hand, it bleeds then a scab begins to form and it heals itself. Secondly, through a miraculous process the body's innate intelligence is put into play.

The Bible speaks of healing for man's body throughout its pages. For instance , in Psalm 103:3, (JKV) the bible says "Who forgiveth all thine iniquities; who healeth all thy diseases;" Jeremiah 17:14 (KJV) says "Heal me O Lord, and I shall be healed, save me and I shall be saved: for Thou art my praise." (1) From a biblical view of this subject matter, one can only trust and believe in the power of the written Word of God; From man's view medically and scientifically, the human body indeed possesses an innate ability to heal itself. If man could believe on the level of receiving the word of God into their hearts concerning this idea of the body's self-healing ability, then walking in divine healing and divine health would cease to be an issue. Often in the process of being healed of a disease or a condition, the mind exerts a powerful influence over the body. In the book of Isaiah 26: 3 (KJV) the Bible says, Thou will keep him in perfect peace, whose mind is stayed on the Lord: because he trusts in thee. It is of the utter most importance that the peace of God is there to keep the body aligned with the Holy Spirit to keep all parts of the body in check. Where the spirit of peace is, according to 1 Peter 5: 7, all cares can be cast upon Him, for He cares for you. So, when spirits of infirmities try to invade the body the spirit of peace steps to the forefront of the mind and allows you to cast that care upon Jesus. Who by the way, " received stripes for our healing." In 1 Peter 2:24, it is stated " who His own self bare our sins in His own body on the tree, that we, being dead to sins, should live unto righteousness; by whose stripes ye were healed." The Great I AM really did provide for man on all fronts. We must believe in the healing power of God. " Now the God of hope fills you with all joy and peace in believing that ye may abound in hope, through the power of the Holy Ghost. (Romans 15: 13) Now if you can abound in hope, you can receive your healing.

CHAPTER 3

FAITH'S ROLE IN THE BODY'S HEALING PROCESS

To all who believe, you must first of all be willing to place all of your faith and trust in the Lord. As we navigate through what is described as faith's role in a journey of the healing process, the word of God's definition of faith is of utmost importance; According to Hebrews 11:1, the Bible says (KJV) " Now faith is the substance of things hoped for, the evidence of things not seen." For without faith it is impossible to please God. And that faith without works is dead. Faith must be acted upon. As your faith grows, you will become more confident in trusting God and believing what He says in His word.

The healing process is described as a journey, because according to the degree of the type of infirmity you are experiencing in your body it may not be an overnight deliverance. As in my own personal experience, one of the journey's involved a recovery process. This particular infirmity was a very stubborn one and God sent His word and healed my body. In the book of Psalm 17:20 it reads, "He sent His word and healed them, and delivered them from their destruction. The word that brought about deliverance for me from that stubborn spirit of infirmity that attached itself to my body came from Psalm 118:17, which says, "I shall not die, but live, and declare the works of the Lord." (KJV) The scripture says, "But it is good for me to draw near to God, that I may declare all thy works, (Psalm 73:28) Whom have I in heaven but Thee? And there is none upon earth that I desire beside Thee. My flesh and my heart fails; but God is the strength of my heart, and my portion forever.(Psalm 73:25-26). He was gracious enough, and loved us enough to give every man a measure of faith. Romans 12:3 says, For I say, through the Grace given unto me, to every man that is among you, not to think of himself more highly than he ought to think, but to think soberly, according as God hath dealt to every man the measure of faith. (Rejoicing in hope, patient in tribulation; continuing instant in prayer.),Romans 12::12.

Our bodies are the temple of the Holy Spirit, so we must work diligently to live healthy lifestyles. Making lifestyle changes involve making a conscientious decision to begin the change by disciplining yourself. The Holy Spirit can really strengthen a person in that area. You won't have to struggle in obtaining the discipline that you need to bring your body and mind under suggestion, just seek the guidance of the spirit and the word.

In many instances in the word of God we can read of people's faith making them whole. For example, "The woman with the issue of blood for twelve years, and had been to see many physicians and spent all that she had and was no better; but rather grew worse; but one day she heard about Jesus, and she pressed her way through the crowd and touched Jesus's garment; The

book of Matthew 9: 20 says, "And, behold, a woman,
which was diseased with an issue of blood twelve
years, came behind Him, and touched the hem of His
garment: For she said within herself, if I may but
touch His garment, I shall be whole. But Jesus turned
Him about, and when He saw her, He said, daughter,
be of good comfort; thy faith hath made thee whole.
And the woman was made whole from that hour.
And because of her faith; straightway the fountain of
her blood was dried up; and she felt in her body that
she had been healed. (KJV) Mark 5: 25-34. When
trusting in God and waiting upon His word to work
for you, your faith will strengthen you because you
are not standing alone, you have taken a stand on the
word of the Living God. The word works, and never
loses its power. There is a verse found in the book of
Jeremiah, 32: 17 which says " Ah Lord God! Behold,
Thou hast made the heaven and the earth by thy great
power and stretched out arm, and there is nothing too
hard for thee. (KJV).

When seeking for or believing to be delivered from a
spirit of infirmity, one must not doubt because of
unbelief; but be strong in faith, giving glory to God,
because without faith it is impossible to please Him.
There are a few verses from the book of Matthew 8:
5-10, that says;

*"And when Jesus was entered into Capernaum, there
Came unto Him a Centurion, beseeching Him,
And saying, Lord, my servant lieth at home sick of the
Palsy, grievously tormented. And Jesus said unto him, I
Will come and heal him. The centurion answered and
said,
Lord, I am not worthy that thou shouldest come under my*

*Roof; but speak the word only, and my servant shall be
healed.*

*For I am a man under authority , having soldiers under
me,*

*And I say to this man, go, and he goeth, and to another,
come*

*And he cometh, and to my servant, do this, and he doeth
it. When*

*Jesus heard it, He marveled, and said to them that
followed, verily I say unto you, I have not found so great
faith, no, not in Israel."*

The healing power of God is a powerful force. It is a
force that brings healing to the body, even after the
doctor shakes his head and says we've done all that
we can do. In many instances , this is when God steps
in and begins.to move according to Ephesians 3: 20
(KJV); " Now unto to Him that is able to do
exceeding abundantly above all that we ask or think,
according to the power that worketh in us; that is
where faith and love intertwines. If you just stop and
think about the unconditional love that God has for
His people, and that His love never runs out. Love
never fails. You can read about unfailing love in
Jeremiah 31:3 (KJV) which says; "The Lord hath
appeared of old unto me, saying, Yea, I have loved
thee with an everlasting love: And because He loves
at all times, think on the fact that His love does not
depend on anything that we have to do to earn it. So
we are able to receive our healing because of the love
that we read about in John 3:16 (KJV) "For God so
loved the world, that He gave His only begotten Son,
that whosoever believeth in Him should not perish,
but have everlasting life; and because of the greatest

love that God has for man, we are already healed according to Isaiah 53:5(KJV) Which says, " But He was wounded for our transgressions, He was bruised for our iniquities: the chastisement of our peace was upon Him; and with His stripes we are healed.

CHAPTER 4

GOD'S PROVISION FOR DIVINE HEALING AND DIVINE HEALTH

Divine means that which pertains to God. Things pass man's ability to figure something out:

" According as His divine power hath given unto us all things that pertain unto life and godliness, through the knowledge of Him that hath called us to glory and virtue: Whereby are given unto us exceeding great and precious promises: that by these ye might be partakers of the divine nature; 11Peter 1: 4-5: (KJV) (excerpt from these two verses):

It is evident that "God" has a plan for man. "For I know the plans I have for you, declares the

Lord, plans to prosper you, and not to harm you, plans to give you hope and a future." (NIV) In His divine wisdom, God had every minute detail planned for man's life here on this earth. He left no stone unturned in providing for our lives." How amazing is our God"?

Divine healing involves God moving supernaturally as He often does in raising a person up from a sickness or disease. God moves best seemingly, in instances where the doctors have reached a standstill in a person's treatment. By exercising faith in God and His word, healing comes to a person in a miraculous way. Many times the physicians will tell a patient that there is nothing else that they can do. That is where man's extremity becomes God's opportunity. Divine healing takes the leading role in the patient's recovery . Miracles take place and supernatural testimonies about the mercy, grace and goodness of God are witnessed and told. So God gets all the glory for you receiving your miracle.

THE POWER OF PRAYER IN THE HEALING PROCESS

The power of prayer often goes beyond mere words that are spoken, but by the spiritual power and belief in what you are asking God for, and that it will be granted. "Therefore I say unto you, What things soever ye desire, when ye pray, believe that ye receive them, and ye shall have them" (Mark 11:24- KJV). When making a request to God for anything, whether to be healed, saved, or simply making a request for a desire of the heart; you must be careful with every word. By prayer and supplication, with thanksgiving, let your request be made known unto God and ye must have confidence that your prayers will be heard by our Father which is in heaven. Always remember that you are praying to your Father, just as Jesus did.

Jesus always knew and had confidence that His Father always heard Him and because He prayed according to the will of His Father, Jesus was always blessed with answered prayer. Remember that we are God's children as well. We are joint heirs with Christ. One of Jesus' disciples said unto Him, "Lord teach us to pray, as John also taught his disciples. Jesus said unto them when ye pray, say, "Our Father which art in heaven, Hallowed be thy name. Thy kingdom come, Thy will be done on earth, as it is in heaven. Give us this day our daily bread. And forgive us our debts, as we forgive our debtors. And lead us not into temptation, but deliver us from evil. For thine is the kingdom, and the power, and the glory, forever. Amen (Matthew 6:9-13-KJV). The Lord's Prayer serves as a pattern for us to pray. But as one grows in the knowledge of the Love of God and faithfulness of our Father which is in heaven. We have come to understand how to pray our own prayers. Reaching out to God in prayer becomes so powerful and spiritual until words can't come close to describing being in the presence of our Lord and Savior. When in his glorious presence you can become illuminated. There you will find fullness of joy, love, and peace that is indescribable.

HEALING THROUGH PRAYER: THE
PRAYER OF FAITH

The Bible says in James 5:14-15 (KJV), " Is any sick among you? let him call for the elders of the church; and let them pray over him, anointing him with oil in the name of the Lord: And the prayer of faith shall save the sick, and the Lord shall raise him up; and if he has committed sins, they shall be forgiven him."

As the church moves from glory to glory, there is a realm of the spirit where we can rise above the spirit of sickness and disease.

In the book of Exodus 15:26 it says, "And said, If thou wilt diligently hearken to the voice of the Lord thy God, and wilt do that which is right in his sight, and wilt give ear to his commandments, and keep all his statutes, I will put none of these diseases upon thee, which I have brought upon the Egyptians: for I am the Lord that healeth thee."

Several times you have read in this chapter and book about infirmities, which are spiritual attacks that can and will come upon the body, and will disguise itself as an illness, and they must be rebuked quickly. Prayer, fasting and taking authority over these attacks of infirmities that come upon the body will cause you to be able to cast them out. You can't afford to allow them to linger, they must be rebuked immediately. An attack of an infirmity comes from Satan himself.

You can read in John 10:10 that says, " The thief cometh not, but for to steal, and to kill, and to destroy: I am come that they might have life, and that they might have it more abundantly."(KJV) People who believe must bless the Name of Jesus at all times, and continually keep His praise in their mouths because the Lord is worthy to be praised. The Bible says, "Let everything that hath breath praise the Lord. Praise ye the Lord." (KJV) As a person, learn how to praise God, and show Him how much He is loved, and how precious He is to them, the more you can gain entrance into His Holy presence. As man's knowledge about God increases, he learns to" pray without ceasing". (1 Thessalonians 5:17) (KJV), and he learns how to pray. There is a question posed in the Bible that ask " Is any sick among you? Let him call for the elders of the church; and let them pray over him, anointing him with oil in the name of the Lord. And the prayer of faith shall save the sick, and the Lord shall raise him up; (James 5:14-15) (KJV)

The power of prayer is amazingly effective, especially when you know and operate in the love and anointing of God. Love is a spiritual force that empowers a child of God in all areas of their Christian life. Your walk with God becomes more effective in every area when you take the time to do what it says in Matthew 11:29, "Take my yoke upon you, and learn of me; for I am meek and lowly in heart: and ye shall find rest unto your souls." Another aspect to remember is that God wants a closer relationship with His children. As a person navigates through this life it is wise to keep your mind staying on the Lord.

It is evident that a person will never know everything about God, but He wants us to learn about Him in receiving revelation knowledge of the time we are living in, gain knowledge on how to love Him, and how to love our fellowman, and how to love ourselves. We therefore learn more about God and how we can gain access to what's available to us by reading the Bible and hearing His spoken words as well. The Lord, Jehovah, will never leave us, nor forsake us. We have the assurance that the Lord will always be there for us, and that promise is based on His unconditional love for man.

When you pray, you must pray with confidence and authority, believing that what you are making a request to God for, you will receive. As you grow in the knowledge of the nature of God and His word, you will understand how powerful prayer can be. Your healing is already paid for by the stripes that Jesus took; (Isaiah 53:5). As you navigate through an emerging life as a prayer intercessor, you will come to an understanding of how to receive your own healing through prayer, and how to pray for those who ask you to pray for their healing as well. So it will not seem like hard labor when we pray, remember that the spirit does the work, we serve as the instruments for God's pleasure.

There are times when a person is beyond being able to find words to pray. In Romans 8:26, the Bible says, "Likewise the spirit also helpeth our infirmities; for we know not what we should pray for as we ought, but the spirit maketh intercession for us with groaning which cannot be uttered. Therefore, because we are spirit filled believers, we have the assistance of the Holy Spirit to help us in times when you feel the pressures of life coming in upon you like a flood. As you grow in the grace of our Lord and Saviour Jesus Christ, you can learn how to pray in the spirit. As you walk in the spirit and the newness of life, you will be able to pray without ceasing. There will be times when you will need an immediate answer to a prayer. Answered prayer can change situations and circumstances that could affect someone's life, maybe even your own. The book of James says "And the prayer of faith shall save the sick, and the Lord shall raise him up;;(James 5: 15).

If you confess your faults one to another, and pray one for another, that you may be healed. The effective, fervent prayer of a righteous man avails much.(James 5:16). There are many instances in the Bible where people received healing through the power of prayer.. For instance in the book of Genesis, (20:17), it is stated that Abraham prayed unto God; and God healed Abimelech, and his wife and his maid servants; In 1Kings13:6, it says, "And the King answered and said unto the man of God, intreat now the face of the Lord thy God, and pray for me that my hand may be restored me again. And the man of God besought the Lord, and the king's hand was restored him again, and became as it was before. Prayer is a powerful resource in seeking God to be healed, and God is no respecter of persons. When you pray, if you believe that you will receive what you are praying for, you will have it. In John 11:40, Jesus said unto Mary, when speaking of Lazarus, "Said I not unto thee, that if thou would believe, thou would see the glory of God? Believers have the authority to operate in the supernatural, and even in a higher realm, which is the glory of God. you must take a stand on the word of God, for your healing, and the healing of others if you are believing for their deliverance. When Jesus received word that he whom thou lovest is sick, speaking of Lazarus, He immediately said, this sickness is not unto death, but for the glory of God, that the Son of God might be glorified thereby. When Jesus saw Mary, and saw that she was weeping. "He said unto her, said I not unto thee that if thou would believe thou shouldest see the glory of God"? That was God's miraculous power manifested, when Jesus raised Lazarus from the dead. In John 11:43(KJV), it is written; "And when He thus had spoken, he cried with a loud voice, Lazarus, come forth. And the Bible says, "And he that was dead came forth, bound hand and foot with grave clothes". Now it is evident that just as Jesus raised Lazarus from the dead, you ought more to believe that God can heal any disease. The power of the gospel far exceeds man's ability to comprehend it.

CHAPTER 5

RECEIVING HEALING BY SPEAKING THE WORD

There is an account in the Bible where Jesus spoke the word and a man at the Pool of Bethesda was made whole.

A MAN HEALED AT THE POOL OF BETHESDA

After this there was a feast of the Jews, and Jesus went up to Jerusalem. ² Now there is in Jerusalem by the Sheep Gate a pool, which is called in Hebrew, Bethesda, having five porches. ³ In these lay a great multitude of sick people, blind, lame, paralyzed, waiting for the moving of the water. ⁴ For an angel went down at a certain time into the pool and stirred up the water; then whoever stepped in first, after the stirring of the water, was made well of whatever disease he had. ⁵ Now a certain man was there who had an infirmity thirty-eight years. ⁶ When Jesus saw him lying there, and knew that he already had been in that condition a long time, He said to him, "Do you want to be made well?"

⁷ The sick man answered Him, "Sir, I have no man to put me into the pool when the water is stirred up; but while I am coming, another steps down before me."

⁸ Jesus said to him, "Rise, take up your bed and walk." ⁹ And immediately the man was made well, took up his bed, and walked.

And that day was the Sabbath. ¹⁰ The Jews therefore said to him who was cured, "It is the Sabbath; it is not lawful for you to carry your bed."

¹¹ He answered them, "He who made me well said to me, 'Take up your bed and walk.'"

The woman with the issue of blood in Matthew 9:20, desired to just touch Jesus's garment, and knew that she would be made whole. She pressed through the crowd moving by faith to get to where Jesus was. With her losing blood, she had possibly become very weak. Even though she had been diseased with that bloody issue for twelve long years, her faith was activated. She gained the strength that was needed to reach out and touch the hem of Jesus's garment. But Jesus turned around, and when He saw her, "He said, daughter, be of good comfort, thy faith hath made thee whole". And the woman was made whole from that hour.

All believers have the same privilege today that the woman with the issue of blood had; You can touch the hem of the spiritual garment of Jesus today. If you will only believe, you can walk and live in divine health because Jesus endured stripes for your healing. The healing power of God is already available and waiting on you to receive it by faith.

Psalms 91:15-16 clearly state the benefits of calling on God in the times of trouble.

15 He shall call upon Me, and I will answer him;
I will be with him in trouble;
I will deliver him and honor him.
16 With long life I will satisfy him,
And show him My salvation."

And it came to pass in those days, that He went out into a mountain to pray, and continued all night in prayer to God. (Luke 16:12; 17-19). And he came down with them, and stood in the plain, and the company of His disciples, and a great multitude of people out of Judea and Jerusalem, and from the sea coast of Tyre and Sidon which came to hear Him and to be healed of their diseases; and they that were vexed with unclean spirits: and they were healed. And the whole multitude sought to touch Him for there went virtue out of Him, and He healed them all. If you are a believer, you can actually live in divine healing and divine health, as well. With divine healing, it can be put into play when a spirit of infirmity, which comes from Satan, attacks your body. Stop it right on the spot by losing the spirit of divine healing. It will put up a defense against that spirit of infirmity (or sickness). You must allow your faith in the finished works of Jesus Christ to flow in the healing anointing. It is very important that we walk by faith and not by sight. According to Habakkuk 2:4, the just, shall live by faith. Every waking moment, our faith should be in operation. Often, when Jesus was healing people, He would say, "thy faith has made you whole." (Matthew 9:22). And sometimes He would say, "according to your faith, be it unto you. So we realize how great a part faith plays in our being healed.

If you were healed by Jesus's stripes, then you must believe the word of God, and use it as a foundational principle to stand on when believing for your healing. God changes not, and His word is forever settled in heaven, "and Jesus answering said unto them, have faith in God, For verily I say unto you, that whosoever shall say unto this mountain, be thou removed and be thou cast into the sea; and shall not doubt in his heart, but shall believe that those things which he saith shall come to pass; he shall have whatsoever he saith. As you navigate through this life, make sure that your faith in God remains operational.

The blessing of a healthy body is directly related to the unconditional love of God. The stripes that were put on Jesus, were for the healing of God's people. He endured the pain because His every thought was about fulfilling the purpose and the will of His Father. In third John 2: , it says, "Beloved, I wish above all things that thou mayest prosper and be in health, even as thy soul prospereth. " So you know that when you pray, you have the confidence that if you ask anything according to His will, He heareth us: And if you know that He heareth us, whatsoever we ask of

Him, we know that we have the petition that we desire of Him. Whatever we ask of God in faith, we shall receive. The only way that you will not receive your petition is that you ask amiss. God honors our prayer request when we ask in faith. It is plainly stated in the word of God that in order for your prayers to be honored by the Lord, you must pray in faith believing that they will be answered favorably. And it is scriptural that faith works by love. So, in order for people to receive their healing from the Lord, they must be operating at all times in the spirit of Love. "Remembering without ceasing your work of faith, and labor of love, and patience of hope in our Lord Jesus Christ, in the sight of God and our Father;" Your faith will grow stronger each day as you go from glory to glory. Your increased faith will enable you to receive the healing that Jesus paid a high price for because He was doing the will of His Father. It is up to us to do the will of our Father.

PRAYER AND FAITH WORKS

As a part of God's Revelation to man of how the healing power of God works, He constantly describes the various methods of how to receive healing through the pages of the bible, which is God's Holy word. He heals in many ways. You should never place limits on God because He can do the impossible. God does work in mysterious ways, His wonders to perform. It is certainly understood that God loves unconditionally and at all times, and He promises to never leave us nor forsake us. So if you can believe

God's word, it will work for you. The bible says, "for
what saith the scripture? Abraham believed God, and
it was counted unto him for righteousness. God's
blessings are upon all who believe, and His word
works. The word of God has always worked for His
people, and serves as a final authority in their lives
bringing victory in any situation.

CHAPTER 6

HEALING BY THE LAYING ON OF HANDS

Many people ask, "Who is qualified to lay hands on the sick?" In the Book of Mark (KJV), 16:17, the Bible says, "And these signs shall follow them that believe; and if you read down further close to the end of the 18th verse of the same chapter you will find where it says, "they shall lay hands on the sick, and they shall recover. So to answer the question in part , of who is qualified to lay hands on the sick, "them that believe ". But with God being God, He is able to work through anyone He desires to. There are people who have the gift of healing. The gift of healing also operates through the Holy Spirit, empowering a person to perform supernatural healing upon certain individuals of faith. Usually a person who operates in the gift of healing is empowered with the healing anointing. The healing anointing comes from God. The healing power of God is transferred to those who first of all have knowledge of God (Jesus) and have faith to believe for their own healing.

James 5:14-15

¹⁴ Is anyone among you sick? Let him call for the elders of the church, and let them pray over him, anointing him *with oil in the name of the Lord. *[15]* And the prayer of faith will save the one who is sick, and the Lord will raise him up. And if he has committed sins, he will be forgiven.*

Unbelief will not allow the healing power of God to work through an individual. And we must be knowledgeable about God and His word, in order to know when the power is present to heal. The healing power of God is transferred to those who have knowledge of God and have faith to believe for their own healing. Unbelief will not allow the healing power of God to work through a person. The Lord does not want us ignorant concerning these things. He wants His people to be knowledgeable about healing, whether it is your own deliverance, or believing for someone else. Healing is available for all who believe and have faith.

Luke 4:40
> *When the sun was setting, all those who had any that were sick with various diseases brought them to Him; and He laid His hands on every one of them and healed them.*

The life that Jesus lived upon this earth serves as an example to every generation of believers to follow. We have the gospel as a guide to lead us to the pattern that Jesus laid. The gospel also serves as a knowledge base to learn more about God And the more that we know about God, and obey His Holy word, the more He will empower us to walk in divine health.

When spirits of infirmity attack the body, don't allow that spirit to linger, rebuke it and take immediate authority over it. God has given believers power over all the power of the enemy, and nothing shall by any means hurt us. As you take full authority, that evil spirit will be driven away by you speaking your healing and standing on the word of God.

The laying on of hands represent one of the many ways that God heals. As man navigates through life, God blesses him to walk in perfect health in order to perform life's daily task. God also gifted doctors to treat the conditions that attack the human body. But man must keep in mind that the doctor treats your condition, but God heals it. In order to fulfill the call of the gospel upon your life, there is a great need for perfect soundness in your body. In the Third Epistle of John, second verse it says, "Beloved, I wish above all things that thou mayest prosper and be in health, even as thy soul prospereth."(KJV) A continued walk of faith will always serve as a bridge to help man cross over into a life filled with peach, love, and joy. And you can experience renewed health on a daily basis focusing on the healing power of God. As the body ages, there are certain changes that will occur, but you must not allow these changes to hinder our work in the ministry or in our daily lives. Remember how the Lord told Moses that his eyesight would not get dim. You must keep in mind that our God is always available to assist us whenever we need Him. He promised to never leave us, nor forsake us. So, as different changes take place in the body, you have the authority to rebuke it, and not receive it. It is important to remember that your healing is already complete. Many stripes were laid upon Jesus for your healing. Now all you have to do is believe and have faith. The latter part of Mark 16:18, says, "they shall lay hands on the sick and they shall recover." Always keep in mind how powerful God's word is. For the scripture says on Hebrews 4:12, " for the word of God is quick and powerful, and sharper than any two edged sword, piercing even to the dividing asunder of soul and spirit, and of the joints and marrow, and is a discerner of the thoughts and intents of the heart." God's word is one of the truths that brings revelation, and then manifestation of what you are requesting from Him. When you are believing for the healing manifestation, you must know that it has already been done in the spirit realm as well as in the natural. It was discussed earlier in this book how God created the body to heal itself. It is also very important that you speak your healing out loud at all times. If someone asks you how you are feeling, tell them that you are feeling just great. According to Romans 4:17, (KJV) and calleth those things which are not as though they were. Sometimes, you may not actually be feeling 100 percent, but you must speak out of your mouth that you are blessed. There may be times when a spirit of infirmity will try to attack your body but you must take immediate authority over that spirit by rebuking it in the name of Jesus. Don't allow those spirits to linger because they will form what is called a stronghold. Drive the devil out by speaking your healing and standing on the word of God. The evil spirit of infirmity will have to flee, because it cannot stand against the power of God because you were already healed.

1 Peter 2:24

"Who his own self bare our sins in his own body on the tree, that we, being dead to sins, should live unto righteousness: by whose stripes ye were healed."

The laying on of hands in order to be healed is one of God's divine purposes for blessing and strengthening our bodies. In order to perform the daily task of life, you need to be in good health. And furthermore, in order to carry out or fulfill the call of the gospel in your life, you need to have perfect soundness in your body. It will make it easier to preach and teach the gospel if your body is in good physical shape.

Don't ever procrastinate when it comes to contending with the devil, because casting him out requires immediate action. All believers have the power to cast out devils in the name of Jesus; and all believers are armed with a heavy duty anointing to operate fully in the power of God. Jesus said, " Verily, verily, I say unto you, he that believeth on me, the works that I do shall he do also; and greater works than these shall he do; because I go unto my Father. To all who believe and have been born again, you have access to the full power of God.

Here you will find examples of people in the Bible who were healed by the laying on of hands. This story begins in Luke 13th chapter and the tenth verse, where it says;

10. And He was teaching in one of the synagogues on the Sabbath.

11. And, behold, there was a woman which had a spirit of infirmity for eighteen years, And was bowed together, and could in no wise lift up herself.

10. And when Jesus saw her, He called her to Him, and said unto her, woman, thou art Loosed from thine infirmity.

11. And He laid His hands on her, and immediately she was made straight, and gloried God.

When a child of God begins to operate in the healing power of God, he/she is automatically catapulted into a higher realm of glory. And when you receive your healing, you are filled with joy and thanksgiving. You immediately get into praise mode with your heavenly Father thanking Him for your deliverance.

Paul receives his sight by the laying of hands in Acts 13:3, " And Ananias went his way, and entered into the house; and putting his hands on him said, Brother Saul, the Lord, even Jesus, that appeared unto thee in the way as thou came, has sent me, that you might receive your sight, and be filled with the Holy Ghost. And immediately there fell from his eyes as though it had been scales. And he received sight forthwith, and arose and was baptized.

Another wonderful account of healing by the laying on of hands is found in the book of Acts 28:8, "and it came to pass that the father of Publius lay sick of a fever and of a bloody flux; to whom Paul entered in, and prayed, and laid his hands on him, and healed him. Publius was chief man of the island of Melita The people of the island of Melita were barbarous people. But the Bible says they showed them kindness. (barbarous- uncivilized, savage, unlettered, ignorant).

There is not one thing that can come upon man that God has not prepared deliverance for. His word alone covers man and brings deliverance. God looked out for His people back in creation, where in the book of Genesis, He said, "it is finished", for all time.(Genesis 2:1-2 "Thus the heavens and the earth were finished, and all the host of them. "And on the seventh day God ended His work which He had made." (finished meaning "brought to perfection).

As God's anointed and chosen ones, we must strive to do God's will just as Jesus did His Father's will. For by one offering, He has perfected forever them that are sanctified. (Hebrews 10:14).

Two blind men healed: And when Jesus departed thence, two blind men followed Him, crying, and saying, thou Son of David, have mercy on us. And when He came into the house, the blind men came to Him; And Jesus said unto them, believe ye that I can do this? They said unto Him, yea Lord. then touched He their eyes, saying, according to your faith, be it unto you. And their eyes were opened: Matthew 9: the same works that Jesus did we can do; And greater works shall we do. "The blind receive their sight, and the lame walk, the lepers are cleansed, and the deaf hear, the dead are raised up, and the poor have the gospel preached unto them.(Matthew 11:5).

It is important that God's people read and study His Holy word in order to know that healing was made available for us by the stripes that were put on Jesus

During His trial. You can read about the cruel things that Jesus endured for man's deliverance. "Who His own self bare our sins in His own body on the tree, that we being dead to sins, should live unto righteousness, by whose stripes we were healed." (1Peter 2:24).

When we pray for our healing, we must believe that we will receive what we are asking for, and expect to receive it. As you grow in the Lord, you will learn how to take authority over any spirit of infirmity that tries to attack your body. Rebuke it in the Name of Jesus, and it cannot stay. It has to go. God gave Jesus a name that is above every name. Jesus' Name is above the name of any disease that has a name, even cancer.

CHAPTER 7

PERSONAL TESTIMONIES

I suffered from a growth on the side of my right breast for over three years. There was no medicine or treatment that helped me to improve. As the growth began to grow, it started to drain a bloody type of fluid. The test didn't actually show that it was cancer. I was given very strong antibiotics, but none of them worked or proved successful in my treatment. One day, I was prompted by God to visit a friend who was a sister in Christ. As a result of that visit, which by the way the Lord had predestined, I received my healing by the laying on of hands by another sister in Christ who was also visiting that particular day. This lady who laid hands on me as I was experiencing this problem proclaimed with a loud voice, "I feel the anointing going up my arm". Then she turned immediately to me and laid her hand upon the place where I was experiencing the growth and I was healed instantly. How great is our God? His ways are indescribable. I gave God praise and glory for divine healing.

Whenever God does something miraculous in our lives, it is very important to turn and glorify His name and say "Thank You Lord". Praise and thanksgiving for all blessings are important to God. In 1Thessalonians 5: 18, the Bible says, "In everything give thanks: for this is the will of God in Christ Jesus concerning you. (KJV)

To understand just how faith works to please God, one must learn the process of walking by faith and not by sight. When you're operating in faith you are able to believe beyond what you see or feel. You take a stand on the word of God." The Lord is the one who heals all of our diseases";(Psalm 103:3 (KJV). At this point, a person who has been healed by God should begin praying to believe for divine healing and then divine health. When we read in the word of God, (the Bible) about all of the miracles performed by Jesus, our faith should be strengthened because we are believers. We believe in the miracle working power of Jesus. If God's people would only believe, nothing would be impossible for them. If you read in Mark 9:23, Jesus said to him, "if" you can only believe, all things are possible to him who believes. (NKJV). Divine healing is available right now. The minute you believe, you can receive divine healing from God. You can open your Bible and read in Luke 5: 12 , about Jesus, and how He went about doing good and healing all manner of sickness and disease. "And it came to pass, when He was in a certain city, behold, a man full of leprosy who seeing Jesus fell down on his face, and besought Him, saying Lord, if thou will, thou can make me clean. And He put forth His hand, and touched him saying, I will, be thou clean. " And immediately the leprosy departed from him.

There was another testimony of how I suffered for many years with a spirit of infirmity in my side. The doctors could never diagnose the exact cause of the pain that I endured. I decided to attend a nearby revival meeting. While in the service on that Monday night, which was the start of the revival, the Evangelist stated at the end of the service that night that he wanted everyone to come back on Tuesday night. He said that God was going to work miracles in the service. I decided to attend the miracle working service on Tuesday night. After the Evangelist had brought a word to the people, he called for anyone who desired prayer to come forward. The Prayer line quickly filled up. After the prayer line was down to about two people, I decided to go up and get prayer for myself. Then, the Holy Spirit said to me " Don't get in the prayer line". So I just sat there. Suddenly the Lord spoke to me and said, "I told you not to get in the prayer line because you are being healed right now". I saw a bright light shine down on me, and felt a heat go through my side. I was divinely healed of the pain that I had suffered for many years.

"Now unto to Him that is able to do exceeding abundantly, above all that We ask or think according to the power that works in us." (KJV) (Ephesians 3:20).

Through faith in the Name of Jesus, people are able to experience perfect soundness in their bodies. If you read in Jeremiah 32:17, where it is prayed," Ah Lord God! Behold, thou hast made heaven and the earth by thy great power and stretched out arm, and there is nothing too hard for Thee:" (KJV). The Lord lets man know that He is their God; "Behold, I am the Lord, the God of all flesh: is there anything too hard for me? (Jeremiah 32:27).(KJV). There is no sickness or disease, no matter how severe, that God cannot heal. How great is our God! how wonderful is our God! Man is required to have faith in God, and place all of their trust in Him. He will never leave us, nor forsake us. God's healing power is always available, and by Jesus stripes we were healed. All that is necessary for man to do is to believe it and receive your healing by faith. Jesus told many of the ones that He healed that their faith had made them whole.

Soundness of the body is important to the servants of the Lord and to all men. The Lord in His divine plan for man let us know that He will restore health unto His people. In 3 John 2,(KJV) He says, "Beloved, I wish above all things that thou may prosper and be in health even as thy soul prospereth". So, it is God's will that man live in good health in order to enjoy all of the benefits that He daily loads us down with.

During the year 2006, I began to feel weak and it seemed as though my energy level was falling lower and lower. My primary care physician had prescribed a monthly B12 injection for me. I stopped getting the injections because I started feeling some better. The weakness and loss of energy started up once more , only it had gotten worse. Around the first of January, 2007, I was diagnosed with a very low iron deficiency. My doctor said once, that I didn't seem to have any iron in my body. She commented that she had never seen it that low on any patient before. She put me on a regime of intravenous iron injections. But the more I received the lower my iron level dropped. The spirit of infirmity that was attacking my body did not let up. She sent me to the hospital in March of 2007. By September of that year, I could no longer walk. After the doctor started speaking death over me, my husband checked me out of that hospital and brought me home. Those doctors said that I had about two weeks to live. My husband had to sign me out due to the seriousness of the condition they say I had. I was extremely weak while at home. I stopped eating and I could not stand to be touched anywhere on my body. My husband went in prayer and the Lord spoke to him about what to do about what I was going through. That was in December 2007. He said the Lord said that I would be going to a hospital in Mississippi. Around the first of January, he carried me to see my primary physician, and she told him that I could not go back home in my condition. She said he could carry me to the hospital or she would call a first responder to carry me. He transported me to the hospital, and the last thing that I remember is being placed on an examining table. The cancer doctors were called in, so was an oncologist for consultation. My hospital stay lasted there a little over three months. I endured six surgeries, and 25 blood transfusions. I thank God that before I had gotten worse that he gave me a verse of scripture to lean on against the attack of the enemy. My verse was and always will be Psalm 118:17; I shall not die, but live, and declare the works of the Lord.

Before I was released from the hospital, I had to take 150 dives in a hyperbaric chamber. Physical therapy came in and started helping me to learn to walk again. It was a process, but God gave me a very speedy recovery. On a Wednesday, one of my husband's cousins came by to see me, and she had a word from the Lord to share with me. She told me that the word was to tell me it was time for me to leave the hospital. I received that word. I was still in a wheelchair, but I immediately told a nurse that I wanted to see my doctor. When He came by that evening to see me, I told him that I wanted to go home. He did not try to keep me any longer, but there were a couple of requirements that he had for me; the first one was to come back for all of my office visits, and the second one was to follow all of the rules that he prescribed for me to follow. It took about six months for my legs to gain strength, but today I am walking and praising God. The Lord manifested my deliverance so quickly in getting me back on my feet again. My blood was fine and so was I. Praise be to the Lord and His amazing healing power. I knew for sure that I was healed of that spirit of infirmity. When God heals, He heals. I am a believer, and I know that God loved me enough to give me a word to stand on in faith. I'm thankful that God prepared a word for me before the foundation of the world, when He said, it's finished.

I was favored by God in another instance when a spirit of infirmity again tried to attack my body.

One evening, I was following the doctor's orders in performing a self-breast exam at home when I discovered two rather large lumps in my right breast. I immediately called my husband and asked him to pray for me. My daughter came into the room as well. My husband prayed a sincere prayer, which is called the prayer of faith in the Bible. The next day I went to the doctor and she examined me and she looked as though she was reluctant to tell me anything. She went out and came back in shortly afterwards, and told me that she had made an appointment in Mississippi with the doctor that performs my mammograms each year. Just before I left the examining room, she told me to be sure and go the doctor the next day and see the other doctor. When I arrived at the doctor's office the next day she examined me and then ordered two mammograms and a biopsy. After viewing the x rays she told me that I would need surgery right away. She said that she couldn't tell me how bad the cancer was, and could I return the next day. She had called a surgeon but the one she called was out of town. My family and I continued in prayer, rebuking the spiritual attack on my body. The next day I arrived at 8:45 A.M. and when the nurse called me back to see the doctor, she said that she had called my house and left a message but I had already left. She looked very puzzled and confused. She said it is not cancer. It looks like you may have obtained some type of trauma or something. I knew that I hadn't but, I heard the spirit of the Lord say, "she couldn't give you her report, until I gave her My report.. I left that office rejoicing along with my husband. When I got home the lumps were still there, and that was not good enough for me. So I said to the Lord, Lord, I want to see your glory, I want you to remove those lumps from my breast. Sometime in the next day or two they were gone. I know that my God is a mighty God. When I read in the Bible how Jesus took those stripes for our healing, I get into praise and worship mode. I pray in the spirit and I now sing in the spirit. I rely on God's word because it works for me. I believe in the healing power of God.

Healing is just one of the many areas of our life that God wants to do great things and show Himself strong in the eyes of His people. Our God is an Almighty God and a loving and kind Saviour. There is one thing that's certain with God, and that is whatsoever it says in His word will work for you, if you believe.

In Isaiah 53:5, it says, "But He was wounded for our transgressions, He was bruised for our iniquities; the chastisement of our peace was upon Him; and with His stripes, we are healed.

Jesus did a wonderful thing for us. He provided forever for our healing, while carrying out the will of His Father. And as a result, we are able to walk in divine health. You will see just how much God loves us when we read in 3 John 1:2 where it says, "Beloved, I wish above all things that you may prosper and be in health, even as your soul prospers." The Lord cares about every area of our lives, He is always near to us. He is our Father and our only hope. I encourage you to place all of your trust in Him. You will discover that He is all you will ever need, He will provide. When we seek Him with our whole heart, we will find Him. He wants us to enjoy good and perfect health. It was a great thing that Jesus did for us. The healing power of God is for real.

Once you learns how to receive your healing, you will be able to take full authority over your body which is

THE HEALING POWER OF GOD

the temple of the Holy Spirit, and rebuke any sickness or infirmity that tries to come upon you. Often, many of God's people will fast and pray until they are free of any attack of Satan to inflict disease upon them. There is an instance stated in the Bible (Matthew 17:21) where Jesus told His disciples: "Howbeit this kind goeth not out but by prayer and fasting." Jesus also informed his people that, " If ye have faith as a grain of mustard seed, ye shall say unto this mountain, Remove hence to yonder place; and it shall remove; and nothing shall be impossible unto you" (Matthew 17:20-KJV). God's people cannot afford to walk in unbelief and expect to receive divine healing because the "just shall live by faith".

In the fourth chapter of the book of Proverbs, the Lord says, "My son, daughter as well, attend to my words; incline thine ear unto my sayings. Let them not depart from thine eyes; keep them in the midst of thine heart. For they are life unto those that find them, and health to all their flesh." God has certainly looked out for His people and provided provision for life upon the earth. He has omitted nothing in His great plan and purpose for mankind. We are His people and the "sheep of his pasture". The shepherd looks out for His sheep, "The name of the Lord is a strong tower: the righteous runneth into it, and is safe (Proverbs 18:10-KJV).

God's people have access to the power that is in the name of Jesus and the power that is in His word. We have all the things that we need to live abundant lives. For we serve a true and living God.

There were many times that I faced sickness (which I call spirits of infirmity) in my body and I was completely ignorant of what to do about it, spiritually. And most of the attacks on my body remained long after many doctor visits. I suffered for many years, struggling with pain and infections, among many others things. I went through many surgeries and blood transfusions, and long hospital stays. Sometimes my body would appear to be healing, only to reactivate the same symptoms. I had accepted Christ in my life in the early 80's and I had the opportunity to meet many of my brothers and sisters in Christ who were going through great trials of affliction in their bodies too. I had been around sickness and disease most of my life, seeing family members suffer until death with no hope in sight. They had not been taught that the God that they served was a healer. Not only that, but His Son, Jesus, endured much pain and turmoil, receiving many stripes with the whip for our healing. Thus, He is called the great physician. "For as much as ye know that ye were not redeemed with corruptible things, as silver and gold, from your vain conversation, received by tradition from your fathers; but with the precious blood of Jesus, as of a lamb without blemish and without spot. Who by Him does believe in God, that raised Him up from the dead, and gave Him glory; that your faith and hope might be in God." (1 Peter 1:18-19) It is very difficult to believe that there were people who attended church and also lived their lives pleasing God, but were not enlightened about the great provision that had been made available for our healing by Jesus Christ. It is now very important to help enlighten people on the blessings of this great and powerful provision of the healing power of God that we have access to.

There is an account in the Bible in Luke 6:19, where it says "And the whole multitude sought to touch Him; for there went virtue out of Him, and healed them all. As you navigate through the pages of the gospel, God will enlighten the eyes of your understanding to gain greater knowledge and insight of the healing power of God. You are to have faith in God. The gospel declares in Mark 11:23-24 that whosoever shall say unto this mountain, be thou removed and be thou cast into the sea; and shall not doubt in your heart, but shall believe that those things which he said shall come to pass, he shall have whatsoever he says. Therefore, what things soever you desire, when you pray, believe that you will receive them, and you shall have them. As you read the Bible, and pray for revelation of God's word, you will begin to understand how the healing process works. In Isaiah 33:24, the bible says "And the inhabitant shall not say I'm sick. The body is often under spiritual attack; so if by Jesus's stripes we were healed, it is conclusive that it is not a sickness but a spirit of infirmity. You must receive God's word as final authority, and it is forever settled in heaven.

AUTOBIOGRAPHY

My name is Carolyn Jones Powe, Prophetess, and I was born in Laurel, Mississippi. My parents later moved to Mobile, Alabama. I am the oldest of my mother's children. I got married to Bishop Lesley Powe on May 5, 1978 to present day. We also have a daughter, LaKeshia Sherell Powe. I have been a minister for over 20 years and I enjoy doing the Lord's work! We all love the Lord and find joy in our work in the Kingdom!

I graduated from Coffeeville High School which is located in Clarke County in Alabama. I attended college at Alabama State University in Montgomery, Alabama, where I earned a Bachelor's degree in Early Childhood Education. I attended graduate school at what was then called Livingston University. Livingston University was later renamed The University of West Alabama. I was a kindergarten teacher at York Westend Junior High School located in York Alabama in the Sumter County school system for over 20 years. God blessed me with a gift to draw out of the kindergarten students their very best learning styles. Many of my former students have become very successful themselves and live successful lives.

In 2011, I founded a nonprofit organization, The Open Door. We operate a food pantry, drive people to doctor's appointments, and a have a Christmas Outreach Ministry. We provide gifts for children.